ILEOSTOMY DIET COOKING TIPS

Natural Food Nutrients

Crafting Your Personal Ileostomy Diet at home

DR. SOFIA SILAS

Table of Contents

CHAPTER ONE

Introduction

Ileostomy surgery may be a life-changing operation for those suffering from inflammatory bowel disease (IBD), colorectal cancer, or other digestive issues.

While it relieves symptoms and improves quality of life, it also causes major changes in food patterns.

Understanding how to handle food and nutrition after ileostomy surgery is critical for overall health and well-being. In this talk, we'll look at the notion of an ileostomy, the necessity of food thereafter, nutritional requirements, and ways for developing a balanced diet plan.

Understanding Ileostomy

An ileostomy is a surgical technique that includes making an incision in the belly and bringing a piece of the small intestine, known as the ileum, to the surface to establish a stoma.

This stoma acts as an alternate route for waste removal when the usual route via the colon and rectum is not working properly.

Ileostomies may be temporary or permanent, depending on the underlying medical problem and the scope of surgical intervention necessary.

The Importance Of Diet Following Ileostomy Surgery

Following ileostomy surgery, patients must adjust to considerable changes in their digestive tract. Because the colon and rectum are bypassed, the ileostomy produces liquid or semi-liquid feces, which may cause issues such as dehydration, electrolyte imbalances, and vitamin shortages if not controlled effectively. As a result, keeping a healthy diet becomes critical to supporting general health and avoiding issues.

Nutritional Needs After Ileostomy

Following ileostomy surgery, the body's capacity to absorb certain nutrients may be impaired. Factors such as lower intestinal surface area and quicker transit time might impact nutrient absorption, necessitating careful dietary choices. Key nutrients that may need particular care are:

1. Monitor and supplement electrolyte levels, especially sodium, potassium, and magnesium, to avoid shortages

and maintain appropriate body functioning.

2. Fluids: Staying hydrated is vital to avoid dehydration, particularly with the increased risk of fluid loss via stoma output. Consuming lots of water and electrolyte-rich drinks may help you stay hydrated.

3. Protein is required for tissue repair and maintenance, especially after surgery. Consuming high-quality protein sources such as lean meats, poultry, fish, eggs, dairy, legumes, and tofu may aid in healing and general health.

4. Vitamins and minerals: Post-ileostomy alterations in digestive function may influence vitamin B12, iron, calcium, and vitamin D levels. Working with a healthcare physician or nutritionist to ensure appropriate intake via food and supplements is critical.

CHAPTER TWO
Navigating Food Options With An Ileostomy

Adjusting to life with an ileostomy entails understanding how various meals affect stoma output and general digestive health.

While no stringent dietary limits exist, some foods may be more prone to produce problems such as increased stool production, gas, or stink. Common triggers include:

1. High-fiber meals, such as fresh fruits and vegetables, whole grains, nuts, and seeds, might be difficult to digest and cause

blockages or excessive stoma output. Cooking or preparing certain meals may make them more palatable.

2. Gas-producing foods: Beans, cabbage, broccoli, onions, and carbonated drinks may cause gas and discomfort. Modifying consumption or choosing fewer gas-forming options might help alleviate symptoms.

3. Consuming spicy or acidic meals, such as citrus fruits, tomatoes, and vinegar, might irritate the digestive system, leading to increased stoma output and pain. It may be useful to

monitor individual tolerance levels and restrict intake of certain foods.

Developing A Balanced Ileostomy Diet Plan

Designing a healthy diet plan after ileostomy surgery entails including a range of nutrient-dense foods while keeping individual tolerances and preferences in mind. Some basic guidelines for developing a healthy ileostomy food plan include:

1. Eating modest, frequent meals may help regulate stoma output and reduce stomach pain.

2.   Maintaining   hydration: Drinking enough of fluids, such as water and electrolyte-rich drinks, is crucial for avoiding dehydration and staying hydrated, especially during hot weather or physical exercise.

3. Including protein-rich meals in every meal helps promote healing, muscular maintenance, and general wellness. Lean meats, poultry, fish, eggs, dairy, lentils, and tofu are all great alternatives.

4. Choose nutrient-dense foods: Consuming fruits, vegetables, whole grains, lean meats, and healthy fats may provide

nutritional demands without causing digestive difficulties.

5. Listen to your body. Understanding how various meals influence stoma output, energy levels, and general well-being may aid in identifying unique triggers and making educated dietary decisions.

To summarize, managing food and nutrition following ileostomy surgery is critical for preserving health, avoiding problems, and promoting general well-being. Understanding the particular problems and nutritional requirements connected with an ileostomy may assist people in developing a well-balanced meal plan that suits their specific needs and preferences. Working closely with healthcare specialists, especially dietitians, may give important advice and support throughout the postoperative period.

Living with an ileostomy has unique problems, especially in terms of food and nutrition. Whether you've just had ileostomy surgery or have been living with one for a long, knowing what foods to eat, what to avoid, and how to manage meals is critical for preserving your health and wellness.

Foods To Include In Your Ileostomy Diet

Maintaining a balanced and healthy diet is crucial for everyone, but it is especially important for those who have an ileostomy. Here are some meals that are typically well-tolerated and useful for people with ileostomies:

1. Choose lean proteins such as skinless chicken, fish, eggs, tofu, and lentils. These meals give the essential amino acids required for tissue repair and general wellness

without producing excessive stool production.

2. Soft fruits, such as bananas, avocados, peeled apples, and ripe melons, are soft on the digestive tract and reduce the risk of stoma obstructions or discomfort.

3. Cooked veggies (carrots, spinach, zucchini, and potatoes) are simpler to digest than raw ones. Steaming or cooking veggies until soft might help relieve intestinal pain.

4. White Grains: Choose refined grains like white rice, bread, and pasta prepared with white flour. These grains are less prone to

irritate or clog the digestive system than whole grains rich in fiber.

5. Consider dairy alternatives for lactose intolerant or sensitive individuals, such as lactose-free milk, almond milk, or soy milk. These options provide calcium and vitamin D without causing intestinal problems.

6. Smooth nut butter, such as almond or peanut butter, provides protein and healthful fats. However, they must be consumed in moderation, since too much fat might cause loose stools.

7. Probiotic Foods: Consuming probiotic-rich foods like yogurt,

kefir, sauerkraut, and kimchi help improve gut health and bowel motions. Probiotics promote a healthy balance of intestinal flora, lowering the risk of digestive issues.

CHAPTER THREE

Foods To Avoid With An Ileostomy

While many meals are safe for people who have an ileostomy, some may aggravate symptoms or create problems. The following foods should be avoided or consumed in moderation.

1. Fibrous meals, such as nuts, seeds, popcorn, raw vegetables, and whole grains, may be difficult to digest and produce stoma irritation or obstructions. Limit your consumption of these items or go for cooked and peeled variants.

2. Gas-Producing Foods: Beans, cabbage, broccoli, onions, and carbonated drinks may cause bloating and discomfort. Monitor your consumption of these items and try eating them in lesser quantities.

3. Spicy and acidic meals, including citrus fruits, tomatoes, and vinegar-based goods, might irritate the digestive system and create pain. These foods should be avoided or consumed in moderation, particularly if you suffer from acid reflux or inflammation.

4. High-fat meals: Consuming greasy or fried meals might increase bowel motions and cause loose stools or diarrhea. Limit your consumption of fatty meals such as fried meats, butter, cream sauces, and fast food to avoid stomach problems.

5. Excess sugar and artificial sweeteners may cause diarrhea and dehydration. Choose natural sweeteners sparingly and study food labels carefully.

6. Tough Meats: Fibrous meat products, such as jerky, may be difficult to chew and digest. To

ease digestion, use soft cuts of meat or other protein sources.

Tips For Cooking And Preparing Meals With An Ileostomy

Cooking and preparing meals with an ileostomy necessitates certain changes to guarantee proper digestion and comfort. Here are a few suggestions to make dinner easier:

1. Chew thoroughly. Take your time chewing food properly to help digestion and limit the possibility of blockages. Avoid taking huge pieces and eat slowly to help your

body metabolize food more efficiently.

2. Stay hydrated. Drink lots of fluids throughout the day to avoid dehydration, particularly if you have increased stool production. Aim for at least eight glasses of water each day and minimize caffeinated or sugary drinks.

3. Monitor portion sizes. Pay attention to portion amounts to avoid overeating, which may strain your digestive system. Eating smaller, more frequent meals throughout the day may aid digestion and reduce pain.

4. Experiment with cooking methods. Investigate alternative cooking techniques such as baking, steaming, or grilling to prepare meals that are simpler to digest. Avoid frying or charbroiling, which may increase fat and cause stomach difficulties.

5. Maintain a food diary to detect trigger foods or digestive habits. This knowledge may help you make more educated decisions and change your diet to properly manage symptoms.

Beverage Options For Ileostomy Patients.

An ileostomy patient's beverage choices are critical to their well-being. Opting for hydrating foods is critical to avoiding dehydration, particularly given the increased risk of fluid loss from the stoma.

Water is the best option for hydration since it replenishes lost fluids without causing stomach problems.

However, electrolyte solutions or sports drinks may help maintain electrolyte balance, especially in hot temperatures or after strenuous exertion. Caffeinated and alcoholic drinks should be avoided since they may cause dehydration and promote gastrointestinal motion, which can be uncomfortable.

CHAPTER FOUR
Managing Hydration With An Ileostomy

Managing hydration with an ileostomy necessitates caution. Individuals must carefully control their hydration intake, particularly in hot weather or during intensive activity.

It is advisable to sip water throughout the day rather than consume enormous amounts all at once.

Additionally, including hydrating items such as fruits and vegetables in the diet might help with total fluid consumption. It is critical to be aware of indicators of dehydration, such as dry mouth, dark urine, or dizziness, and to refill fluids immediately.

Understanding Food Labels For The Ileostomy Diet

Understanding food labels is critical for ileostomy patients to maintain good digestive health. Paying attention to fiber level is critical, since high-fiber diets may cause digestive system obstructions.

Choosing low-fiber options or fully cooking fibrous veggies may help reduce this risk. Monitoring sugar and fat levels is also important, since some meals may aggravate digestive problems or lead to weight gain. Reading labels carefully and selecting meals that are readily digested might help you feel more comfortable and healthy.

Eating Out With An Ileostomy: Tips And Strategies

Dining out may be difficult for those with an ileostomy, but with good preparation, it can be a pleasant experience. Researching restaurant menus ahead of time helps you to choose items that meet your dietary restrictions and tastes. When ordering, suggest steaming veggies instead of raw or grilled meats without strong sauces to reduce gastric pain.

Bringing additional supplies, like as pouches or wipes, ensures that you are prepared for any unanticipated scenarios. Furthermore, disclosing dietary requirements or preferences to restaurant workers may help ensure a more accommodating eating experience.

Social And Dining Etiquette With An Ileostomy

Maintaining dignity and comfort while socializing and eating with an ileostomy is critical. Open communication with friends and family about food preferences and restroom accessibility may reduce tension and guarantee a pleasant social experience.

When attending a meeting or function, quietly finding the toilet upon arrival may bring comfort and peace of mind. It is critical to emphasize self-care and avoid feeling obligated to ingest meals or drinks that may cause pain. Individuals may confidently and easily navigate social settings by arguing for their own needs and limits.

Navigating Special Occasions With An Ileostomy

Special events often concentrate on food, which presents special complications for those who have an ileostomy. Planning and talking with hosts about dietary limitations or preferences may assist ensure that appropriate alternatives are available.

Bringing snacks or meals that are both safe and pleasurable to eat will help you feel more in control and included. It is critical to concentrate on the company and celebration rather than just the food, stressing the social side of the event. Individuals who approach special occasions with flexibility and a positive mentality may fully participate while managing their nutritional demands.

To summarize, beverage choices, hydration control, food labeling comprehension, eating out tactics, social etiquette, and managing special events are all important parts of living a healthy and meaningful life with an ileostomy. Individuals who prioritize self-care, communication, and readiness may easily manage a variety of food and social circumstances, preserving their health and satisfaction.

CHAPTER FIVE
Traveling With An Ileostomy:
Dietary Considerations

Traveling may be a wonderful experience, but for people with ileostomies, it can also provide unique obstacles, particularly in terms of food restrictions.

An ileostomy, a surgical operation that creates a hole in the belly to divert digestive waste, necessitates strict control over what enters the body to guarantee comfort and good health when on the move.

Dealing With Digestive Problems: Tips And Remedies

Due to alterations in bowel function, people with ileostomies often have digestive problems. However, there are a few ideas and cures that may help relieve pain and preserve regularity.

It is critical to remain hydrated by consuming enough of fluids, particularly water, to avoid dehydration and help digestion. Fiber-rich meals, such as fruits, vegetables, and whole grains, may also aid with bowel motions. Furthermore, integrating probiotics into the diet may improve gut health and alleviate symptoms such as bloating and gas.

Coping With Food Allergies And Intolerances

Food allergies and intolerances might complicate nutritional management for those who have an ileostomy. To avoid unpleasant reactions, identify and avoid trigger foods.

A meal journal may help monitor symptoms and identify harmful items. Working closely with a healthcare physician or a nutritionist may also give individualized advice and assistance for properly managing food allergies and intolerances.

Mindful Eating Strategies For Ileostomy Patients

Mindful eating entails focusing on the sensory experience of eating, which includes flavor, texture, and enjoyment. Mindful eating may benefit ileostomy patients by improving digestion and reducing pain. Chewing food fully and eating slowly may help digestion and lower the likelihood of blockages.

It's also important to watch food amounts and prevent overeating, which may strain the digestive system. Planning meals ahead of time and selecting nutrient-dense foods will help you achieve a balanced diet that promotes overall health and well-being.

Staying Positive And Motivated During Your Ileostomy Diet Journey

Maintaining a good attitude and being motivated are critical components of effectively managing an ileostomy diet, particularly while traveling. It is critical to concentrate on what may be enjoyed rather than obsessing over dietary limitations. Exploring new foods and dishes that meet your dietary demands may make the experience more pleasurable.

Connecting with people who have gone through similar circumstances, whether via support groups or online forums, may also be encouraging and inspiring. Celebrating accomplishments, no matter how minor, may increase morale and maintain good behavior.

Conclusion

Traveling with an ileostomy necessitates careful dietary choices to promote comfort and well-being while on the road. Individuals may confidently and easily manage their ileostomy diet journey by treating digestive concerns with practical suggestions and cures, dealing with food allergies and intolerances, practicing mindful eating, and having a happy mentality.

With appropriate preparation and assistance, traveling with an ileostomy may be a rewarding experience that adds to life's experiences.